AMERICAN
HYGGE

*How You Can Incorporate Coziness Into Your
Living Space and Bring Warmth to Your
Relationships Without Moving to Denmark*

By

Melanie Morgan

advice. The content within this book has been derived from various sources. Please consult a licensed professional before attempting any techniques outlined in this book.

By reading this document, the reader agrees that under no circumstances is the author responsible for any losses, direct or indirect, which are incurred as a result of the use of information contained within this document, including, but not limited to, — errors, omissions, or inaccuracies.

ISBN: 9781729075265

Table Of Contents

Chapter 1: Introduction..1

What is Hygge, and Where it Comes From 1

The Origins of Hygge 2

Acquiring the Hygge Mindset 2

Transform a Lonely Night into a Respite for the Weary Soul 5

Hygge vs. Minimalism...6

How Hygge and Minimalism Fit Together 6

So Let's Start with Minimalism 6

Now Let us Move onto Hygge…......................................7

Hygge can be a Natural Extension of Simplicity 7

There is More to Minimalism and Hygge than Material Things...8

Bringing Hygge and Minimalism into Your Home 9

Slowing Down..12

It is the Simple Things that Matter 13

1. Be in the Present...14

2. Have Quality Time with Family and Friends 14

3. Light Up the Candles...15

4. Create a Comfortable Space....................................15

5. Step Outside 16

6. Fall in Love with Food 17

7. Take Some Break..17

Hygge and Gratitude..18

Create that Cozy Atmosphere 18

Have Your Self-Care Kit Around 19

Learn a Craft...19

Make a Hygge Meal...20

Start a New Tradition with Your Loved Ones.................20

Gratitude is an Art. Practice it 21

Chapter 2: Hygge and Home Décor 23

So How Do You Hygge?.......................................23

Hygge Décor Tips for Your Home 24

    1. Adopt Neutral Color Schemes................25

    2. Create a Comfortable Atmosphere.....................25

    3. Bring in the candles....................................26

    4. Light up those areas with twinkly lights.................26

    5. Make a fire..27

    6. Throw in some texture...............................27

    7. Hygge for every season 28

    8. Less is more when it comes to Hygge 28

Chapter 3: Hygge and Your Wardrobe 29

    1. Oversize it 29

    2. Street Style Fleece 30

    3. It is All About the Fabric.............................30

Hygge Fashion Tips for Men.................................30

    1. Get Knitting..32

    2. Go for Muted Colors 32

    3. Bring the Beanies Back 33

    4. Tight is Not Right..33

Hygge Fashion Guide for Ladies..33

   1. Love Everything Knitted 34

   2. Accessorize for the Weather 35

   3. Protect your Eyes 35

   4. Invest in Muted Hues 35

   5. Give Up the Heels 36

Chapter 4: Hygge, Food, and Drink 37

Simple Rules for Eating Together the Hygge Way 37

Suppose Hygge was a Taste, Would it be Kokumi?......39

Making Room for Imperfection...40

What this Means..40

Hygge, Health, Wellness, and Indulgence 41

What this Means for You..41

Some Takeaways...42

Chapter 5: Hygge and Relationships 43

   1. They Value a Cozy Home...44

   2. They Do Not Come Home with the Drama 44

   3. They do not get into debt to fund their
      weddings…..45

   4. Danes are Intentional about the Time They Spend
      Together...45

   5. They Know How to Enjoy the Small Things
      Together…..46

   6. They are the Masters of their Own Traditions.........46

   7. Their Divorces are Less Nasty 47

Building a Healthy Relationship with Hygge...................47

   Communication..48

   Connection..49

Collaboration...51

11 Helpful Ways to Practice Hygge as a Family............53

Decide to Make it a Point, Not an Accident............53

Create Comfortable Meeting Places.......................53

Go Technology Free..54

Be in the Present...54

Cook Together...55

Play Board Games..55

Check Out those Old Photos.....................................56

Wear Comfortable Clothes.......................................57

Get Hot Drinks...57

Do Not Prepare the Agenda....................................58

Hygge and Parenting..59

Independence is Important for Children.......................61

Encouraging Intentional Time..61

A Regular Sabbath is Essential.......................................62

Chapter 6: Hygge Throughout the Year..........65

Hygge for Winter..65

Hygge and Spring..67

Hygge and Summer...68

Hygge and Autumn...70

Hassle-Free Hygge Ideas for the Year...........................71

Chapter 7: Hygge and the Workplace............73

1. Power in Numbness..73

2. Practice Mindfulness in the Workplace..................74

3. Take Coffee Time Seriously.......................................74

4. Shower Your Workspace with Some Love.............75

5. Be Nice...75

Even if You Live in a Warm Climate, You can still
Embrace Hygge...75

1. Come to Work with Your Mug 76

2. Create a Relaxing Work Playlist 77

3. Have Your Lunch Outside or Take Some Time to
Unwind with Colleagues..77

4. Decorate Your Desk or Workspace 78

5. Organize a Potluck with Coworkers 78

6. Embrace Random Acts of Kindness for Your
Colleagues...79

7. Embrace Teamwork 79

8. Learn to be Calm and Content...............................80

The Hygge décor and Your Workplace: The Employer's
Role...81

Smart Casual is Cool… 83

Hygge: The Culture of Togetherness................................83

Make Hygge the Frame of Mind…..................................84

Hygge during Lunchtime...85

Hygge at Home, Happy at the Work...............................85

Hygge Treats...86

Chapter 8: Hygge on a Budget....................................... 87

1. Clearly Understand What You Need 87

2. Buy Used Items...88

3. Shop at the Discount Store 88

4. Create a Hygge Fund 89

5. Start with One Hygge Space 89

Simple Tips to Hygge on a Budget 90

Stay at Home 90

Include a Flagship Mug in Tour Collection 90

Embrace Fire 91

Get crafty 91

Read more 91

Do not give up cooking delicious meals 92

Find indulgence in small pleasures 92

Chapter 9: Getting Started with Hygge 93

Start Taking Time Out 93

Think Introvert 94

Embracing the Hygge Self 95

Simplicity is Key 96

It is the Little Pleasures 97

Create time for friends and family 98

Multi-Tasking is Against the Spirit of Hygge 98

Leave Work at a Reasonable Time 99

Eat Well 99

Wear Comfortable Outfits 100

Conclusion 101

Bonus 102

CHAPTER 1

INTRODUCTION

What is Hygge, and Where it Comes From

Hygge (pronounced hoo-gah) is a popular Danish concept that involves embracing warm feelings that are facilitated by a cozy environment and good company. It loosely translates into "wholesome wellness." Defining hygge in one sentence can be difficult since it is more about a collection of factors that work together to create a cozy and inviting environment.

Hygge goes far in illuminating the soul. Ideally, hygge is meant to create a warm atmosphere while enjoying the good things that life has to offer. Watching a movie with someone special? That is hygge. Hot chocolates and down blankets? That is hygge. The inviting glow of a candlelight? Well, that is hygge too! There is nothing more hygge than being together with family and friends, discussing the small and big things in life. Perhaps this could be the secret as to why Danes are some of the happiest people on earth!

The Origins of Hygge

Hygge's origin is not in the Danish language but rather in the ancient Norwegian, where it loosely translated into "well-being." It was first used in the Danish language towards the end of the 18th century and the Danes have never let go of it. One beautiful thing about hygge is that you can apply it just about everywhere, and the Danes generously allocate it in everything that is commonplace.

Acquiring the Hygge Mindset

Winter can be a long, sluggish season, especially when you live in the land of thick snow. These months of the year can be dark for weeks on end, with sub-zero temperatures and unending winds that bite to the bone. It is natural to look at winter as a season to endure, a time of year to hibernate and barely survive, and hope against hope that your toes will eventually somehow warm back up again.

And no matter how often you give winter a cold shoulder, it continues to visit year after year! And this is where a new approach comes in; a shift in mindset to train yourself to cease slogging along and make winter months more joyous than ever. With that, it is time to try hygge. According to Danes, hygge is a sensibility of togetherness, intimacy, warmth, and well-being. In other words, hygge is the embodiment of that feeling you experience around Christmas time when everything has a sense of a magical glow around it and when everyone you love is around – the only thing is that hygge is applied all throughout the year, and not just during Christmas time!

A word with a powerful meaning, hygge is a lot like an abstract concept that you can apply to countless aspects of your life. Creating a hygge environment where you live can help you wade through the challenges of winter, whether by walking through the freshly fallen snow, inviting family and friends for a dinner party, curling up with your favorite book and a cup of hot coffee, or going to the local rink for ice skating. In that coziness, you can pause and marvel the beauty of life and find happiness and fulfillment from unexpected sources.

With the hygge mindset, you can begin to practice gratitude everywhere you go, even if you are not comfortable with your surroundings. That change in attitude is something you can apply long after winter. You can take it with you in all the seasons throughout life when you are discouraged by a family or a relationship situation, dissatisfied with your job, or frustrated by the situations in your life.

By embracing hygge, you can make every moment in life meaningful and learn how to best take care of yourself. When you embrace hygge, a night out with friends changes from a couple of drinks to blow off steam after a long workday to an evening with people you love, talking about things that truly matter to you. Hygge can transform a boring evening into a respite for troubled souls, with coffee and books being just the balm you need to revive after a tough week. It is seeing a candle as a little ray of hope through the cold, dark night.

Transform a Lonely Night into a Respite for the Weary Soul

Hygge is not just a feeling you get when life is bright and happy. It is a mindset you develop that helps you see the bright and happy when things are not going your way. While it may not dispel your present difficulties, it can help offload some of the heaviness.

So, wherever you find yourself today, whether in an emotional darkness or in the throes of an actual winter, you do not have to stop holding your breath until the season is over and the flowers start to bloom again. Rather, focus on finding joy and fulfillment, wherever you are. You can either fight these seasons or opt to embrace them...and life will always be warm and gentle when you decide to embrace it.

Hygge vs. Minimalism

How Hygge and Minimalism Fit Together

Since hygge is all about slowing down to appreciate life's simple moments, it is easy to understand how minimalism and hygge blend together.

So Let's Start with Minimalism

Minimalism is all about making a decision on what is for keeps, then getting rid of everything else that is not essential or is distracting you from what is essential. Minimalism lets you free your life of clutter, busyness, and distractions from your life. It empowers you to slow down and simplify your life, so you can create more time and space to focus on appreciating the people, things, and activities that you love.

You create more time and space in your life when you opt to slow down and own less material. The result is mindful living, giving yourself the opportunity to appreciate, and be present for the people and things you love most.

Now Let us Move onto Hygge...

Hygge takes simplicity further by encouraging you to savor and draw satisfaction from simple, everyday occurrences. Hygge empowers you to slow down, be available, make connections, and find happiness in those simple daily moments. Hygge gets you to appreciate the simple, cozy moments in your life where you can find joy and gratitude.

Hygge can be a Natural Extension of Simplicity

Both minimalism and hygge work towards creating a space that you love. Both are about intentionally creating your living space and filling it with the people and things you love. This allows you to create a space where you will feel happy and fully enjoy. You will not be distracted by piles of unnecessary clutter. Instead, your home will feel warm and inviting in a simple and clutter-free way.

Removing the clutter, excesses, and distractions are key to creating an inviting space that is easy to enjoy. All you have to do is be clear about the things you value and what is essential for you. Besides helping you create a more simplified, minimalist home, it also makes it easy for you to begin incorporating more hygge to your days.

There is More to Minimalism and Hygge than Material Things

It is important to understand that hygge is not about material things. You do not have to own or buy anything to embrace hygge. Rather, it is about finding satisfaction and contentment and being available for the simple, day-to-day moments of your life; and figuring out how to celebrate those moments.

You do not have to buy anything or introduce anything into your home to embrace hygge. Rather, hygge is all about creating an environment where you feel present rather than preoccupied or stressed by tons of clutter - an environment where you are glad to slow down, relax, and enjoy the simple things of life. Both hygge and minimalism promote contentment with what you have – acknowledging that it is the simple moments in life that make sense in the long run.

Although minimalism initially feels very much about material things as you get to declutter what you do not need, at its core, minimalism has a very little to do with material things. It is about simplicity, so you can create time and space for greater experiences and more fun with doing what you love.

Hygge and minimalism encourage you to be intentional with your space and time so you can focus and be mindful of the important aspects of your life. They help you create a welcoming home that you love and are delighted to welcome others into. Both hygge and minimalism work towards letting you create connections and memories without having to worry about the tons of clutter in your home.

Bringing Hygge and Minimalism into Your Home

When creating your hygge, minimalist home, it is important that you focus on creating a space that you love and enjoy spending time in, and are proud to invite others into.

When you bring your minimalist spin on, incorporating more hygge into your living space and life becomes less about the stuff you need to bring in and more about creating an ambiance and a home that you will enjoy. It becomes a matter of creating a living space you love and can fill with joy, memories, and special moments, not stuff.

The first step to incorporating minimalism and hygge into your living space is getting rid of the clutter. Clutter creates lots of unnecessary distraction. Instead of a relaxing, cozy, and comfortable living space, too much clutter is bound to leave you stressed, overwhelmed, and unable to enjoy life. Eliminate clutter and distractions, and only leave things that you love and are able to bring joy into your life.

Keep in mind, less is more when bringing coziness into your living space while keeping it simple. It is perfectly fine to keep things that bring coziness to your living space. Just be sure to keep it simple and avoid bringing in unnecessary clutter.

Few examples of how you can incorporate hygge into your living space while still keeping it simple:

⇨ Clear your home of decorative clutter. In place of decorative clutter, decorate your home instead with items that bring you happiness while personalizing your living space.

⇨ Get rid of clutter and distractions from your home so you can dedicate more time to the people and things you love.

⇨ Create more time to connect and spend time with loved ones. Cuddle up, play games, read, relax with a cup of coffee or wine together as you talk about what really matters.

⇨ Dim the lights and light up the candles. Candlelight has a special way of bringing in the ambiance and creating a cozy atmosphere for your home. Keep clutter away by avoiding the temptation to pile up too many candles. You can also introduce lamps and twinkle lights alongside the candles to create different light intensities.

⇨ Create a relaxed environment. Play your favorite soft music, prepare your cup of coffee or glass of wine, switch off your phone and just be available!

⇨ Thoughtfully prepare your meals, then set aside enough time to enjoy it. Sharing a room with family and friends is a great way to incorporate even more hygge.

All these tips are quite easy to adopt when you first declutter and simplify your home. You create more space and time in your living space and life when you are not preoccupied with stuff. Instead, minimalism allows you to appreciate these simple hygge moments.

Slowing Down

Hygge is all about being in and enjoying life's every moment, the mindful appreciation of simple things like friends, food, music, and hobbies. Hygge has nothing to do with buying the most expensive candle and stuff from your favorite store. Hygge is appreciating the beautiful warmth of candlelight in the night.

It is the Simple Things that Matter

The beauty of hygge lies in its ability to create pleasure out of the simple things in life. It is about finding comfort in a well-prepared cup of coffee, lighting candles at the dinner table, and inviting friends and family over to share a meal. It is taking a step back from a long week to relax, breath, and appreciate the moment. The Danes have crafted this art into a lifestyle. While it is painfully cold most of the year, their homes are designed to create an inviting warmth and comfort with fabrics and textiles, furniture, and designs.

Wellness is about creating a strong rapport between yourself and the world around you.

Hygge strengthens this rapport through nurtured responsiveness, consideration, and delight in relationships with loved ones. You cannot find hygge in objects or styles, but rather in connections that you let into your life.

Here are seven tips to slowing down with hygge:

1. Be in the Present

The philosophy of hygge is slowing down to enjoy life's precious moments throughout the day. Yes, striking a balance between work and family can be tough; however, there are opportunities to sit back and rest, whether when making your cup of coffee, catching up with a loved one over lunch break, or taking time to think through and appreciate the simple blessings that make life worth living. If you only have one hour to spare, you can still light up a candle, grab a cup of coffee, and read a chapter of your favorite book. In acknowledging the limitations that life throws your way, and in knowing that you have control over your attitude in any given circumstance, you will be able to make the best out of every situation.

2. Have Quality Time with Family and Friends

In this era of life on a first lane, it is pretty easy to lose touch with loved ones. In fact, most have lost the comfort and truthfulness of the actual and literal, and the need to connect. Hygge outlines a way of being that reintroduces warmth and humanity back into the home, workplace, school, and environment. Hygge originates from a society that focuses on people rather than material things. It is powered by the language of love, and to the concept that real wealth lies not in what you accumulate but rather what have and are willing to share.

3. Light Up the Candles

In case you do not know, the Danes have one of the highest candle consumption figures in the world! And this is because the Danes just absolutely love candles. Lighting up the candle, dimming down the lights, and creating an ambiance of warmth and softness is at the core of hygge. Light your candles first thing in the morning, or at night when having dinner with your family. Turn off all the lights and create a serene atmosphere with lots of flickering candlelight.

4. Create a Comfortable Space

Creating a hygge home starts by furnishing your living space with the fabrics you love, enjoy touching, and spending time with. Your home should be designed for solitude and participation, sociability, privacy, and stillness. At the end of the day, it is about that blanket throw over the couch and comfortable slippers.

5. *Step Outside*

While most people associate hygge with indoor moments during the freezing winter months, blanket and slippers, and a burning fireplace, the Danes adapt it all year round. This means stepping out to enjoy the outdoors as well, in any weather. To the Danes, hygge is also about cycling through the city, wrapped in scarves and meeting and greeting family and friends. It is grabbing that picnic gear and heading outdoors during those warm months to enjoy the warmth on the face and skin. Why not embrace the outdoors by strolling around your neighborhood, adding plants to your home, and spending some time tending your garden? Nature is an instrumental part of hygge and, according to experts, should be embraced to fully reap the benefits of this lifestyle.

6. *Fall in Love with Food*

Cooking and sharing meals is another fundamental pillar of hygge. By practicing this on a routine basis, you will naturally find yourself slowing down and enjoying the process. Invite a family or friend to your kitchen and bake a loaf from scratch or batch some biscuits to fill your home with that aroma that comes with baking. Remember, food cooked and shared in love is central to human nature. Sharing a meal is a hallmark of hygge as this brings people together, nourishing both bodies and spirits.

7. *Take Some Break*

Switch off the TV or put down that phone. It is hard to embrace hygge when you are constantly browsing your social media pages. So many people are glued to the virtual world of connectivity. While hygge is not a life free of technology, it advocates for a balance of commitments. It stresses the value of conversation, interactions, and physical intimacy. Hygge is meant to liberate you to fully dwell at the moment without feeling the pressure to record it.

Hygge and Gratitude

The Danes, despite their long, freezing-cold winters, are considered the happiest people on earth. The reason? They are simply grateful of the little things that life has to offer. Hygge is all about "coziness of the soul" with its key ingredients being relaxation, togetherness, indulgence, presence, and comfort. Think of a hug, without physical contact. The key to hygge lies in appreciating and making the most out of the little, daily pleasures, especially during those chilly winter months. Here are six tips for incorporating more hygge into your daily life with a touch of gratitude.

Create that Cozy Atmosphere

Danes are passionate about interior design because it will become their homes – or their hygge headquarters! The one thing every hygge home cannot do without is a "hyggekrog"- that cozy nook that lets you enjoy your coffee and a book. You can also add hygge to your living space through the use of a candlelight, rich textures, and nature. Danes tend to bring the entire forest indoors – branches, leaves, animal skins, fruits, nuts - you name it!

Have Your Self-Care Kit Around

Instead of returning home after a long day and ranting out on social media, why not try a self-care ritual that boosts the R&R that is wearing you down? This is where creating a self-care kit with comfort items like chocolate, candles, coffee, a soft blanket, woolen socks, and your novel or photo album comes in. This self-made kit can greatly help you wind down in a mindful way while expressing gratitude for life's simple things.

Learn a Craft

Knitting is a great hygge since it is a slow, systemic rhythm that calms most people. It can help you focus in a laid-back way. However, if knitting is not your thing, then there are tons of other hygge past-timers you can adopt. Crafts are generally hygge, especially if you can team up with a friend for one. This is a time to slow down and create something with your own hands. You can try painting, quilting, or making a collage in the evening or over the weekend.

Make a Hygge Meal

Hygge foods are all about bringing pleasure. From cakes to cookies, and pantries, Danes love it freshly baked. And remember, it does not have to look professional – in fact, the more rustic, the greater. A slow, rich home-made food like stew and chili is a great hygge. And even more hygge than eating these foods is preparing them with a loved one. Consider ditching those traditional dinner parties for cooking clubs. You maximize the hygge when family and friends gather and cook together rather than one person hosting the party. This is more relaxing and fulfilling, letting you appreciate the people in your life.

Start a New Tradition with Your Loved Ones

Togetherness is an important component of the hygge concept. To create more time with loved ones, consider coming up with a new past-timer that involves a hygge activity – something that encourages everyone to belong and feel comfortable. This could be a game night, cabin rental, ski trip, or apple picking. A meaningful activity that unites the group will certainly knit everyone more tightly together over time. Hygge is making the most of the present, but it is also a way of getting together and celebrating happiness. Danes traditionally plan for hygge moments and reminiscence about them thereafter.

Gratitude is an Art. Practice it

Hygge and gratitude are inseparable. The concept entails feeling grateful for the little things like a cup of hot coffee, or a bike ride on a bright day, or reading your favorite movie. Studies show that grateful people are not only happier but are also less materialistic, more forgiving, and helpful. Hygge is all about savoring simple pleasures.

CHAPTER 2

HYGGE AND HOME DÉCOR

Hygge can best be described as enjoying the simple pleasures of life. While this word is meant to define the Danish way of life, it also defines their décor. The primary idea of hygge décor is creating a peaceful, serene living space that is devoid of clutter. Clutter can be stressful, which negates the concept of the calm and happy way of the Danish lifestyle. While the hygge concept is largely associated with winter, it can actually be enjoyed all year round. In this section, you will learn how to hygge, simple tips, and a few hygge décors do's and don'ts.

So How Do You Hygge?

Hygge is the Nordic way of life that spreads calm and warmth. It appreciates health and happiness and can be realized in many ways. Here are a few ways that you can introduce hygge into your lifestyle:

- ⇨ Surround yourself with the people you love

- ⇨ Appreciate the simple pleasures

- ⇨ Live in the present and be thankful

- ⇨ An extra hour in bed does not harm

- ⇨ Take up a new hobby

- ⇨ Learn to reuse and recycle

- ⇨ Barbeque outdoors

- ⇨ Avoid stress

- ⇨ Enjoy a good movie or book

- ⇨ Appreciate the surrounding

Hygge Décor Tips for Your Home

Hygge's philosophy is all about creating a safe and lively space for family and friends. While decorating, be sure to keep things as simple as you possibly can in order to immerse yourself in this carefree and cozy lifestyle. Here are eight ways you can incorporate a hygge in your living space.

1. *Adopt Neutral Color Schemes*

Your home décor's color scheme should never be too overwhelming when it comes to hygge. Every décor you introduce into your home should contribute to an atmosphere of peace and harmony. Sticking with neutral colors is vital when creating a relaxing space. You can create a comfortable space with pastels colors like light grays, creams, and browns.

2. *Create a Comfortable Atmosphere*

Coziness is the name of the game when it comes to hygge décor. One way to achieve this is by decorating your home with soft comforters and fluffy pillows. Cuddle up on the couch with your blanket and pillows as you unwind after a long day at work. You can also achieve this by creating beautiful nooks like a love seat or window bench. These make for an excellent place to relax with your favorite music or a cup of coffee for the much needed peace of mind.

3. Bring in the candles

What comes into mind when you think of candles? Perhaps a romantic dinner, a calm night with your favorite book, or a relaxing bath. These are the telltale features of the Hygge philosophy. You can never replace the soft and kind candle glow with anything. Create a warm ambiance in your home using candles.

4. Light up those areas with twinkly lights

Twinkly lights are also excellent when creating your hygge décor. Besides being cheery and festive, they also look perfect just about anywhere. You can have them in your living room, bedroom, or even on the outdoor patio. Like candles, twinkly lights produce a soft light and can bring a pleasant touch to your home without going overboard.

5. *Make a fire*

In Danish culture, family and friends gather around the fire to have quality time together. This hygge concept brings togetherness and warmth and is guaranteed to give any home a cozy and welcoming experience. This also ties up to the third and fourth points which are lighting. Introducing layers of light, such as twinkle lights, candles, and fire brings an incredible home feeling in your hygge décor. Sitting around the fire is such a heartwarming concept that you should embrace pretty much every day.

6. *Throw in some texture*

To most people, the texture is not the first thing that comes to mind when they think about a cozy hygge décor. However, incorporating texture into your living space is a great way of adding flavor to an otherwise minimalist design. You can achieve this by warm, natural materials like wool and wood into your décor. You can also incorporate variety by introducing different kinds of colors for a small pop of color.

7. Hygge for every season

By now, you should appreciate that you can adapt hygge as a life style throughout the year. Candlelit nights, coffee, home baked bread, time with family and friends, a soak in the sun – you can enjoy all these without introducing the season factor. You can also organize a bonfire, barbeque nights, or dinner parties. The point is, there are plenty of options if you want to embrace the spirit of hygge and spend quality time with loved ones.

8. Less is more when it comes to Hygge

Start by getting rid of the stuff you are no longer using from your home. Remove everything that no longer serves a purpose because they are only cluttering and crowding your living space. Purchase furniture and décor according to your home's size. If your living room is small, then keep things as minimal as possible.

CHAPTER 3

HYGGE AND YOUR WARDROBE

Rooted in the Nordic culture that takes comfort in the daily beauty of life's little moments, the hygge-inspired lifestyle can last through the year. While minimal living, candles, and connectedness are essential components of a hygge-focused lifestyle, when it comes to the wardrobe, drape fabrics, oversized knits, and neutral hues are also indispensable.

Here are a few key pointers that can help you keep your wardrobe hygge-inspired.

1. Oversize it

One aspect of hygge you can never overlook is the cozy comfort. As the chillier weather sets in, consider keeping the sentiment going strong with a baggy cardigan made from wool or lighter knit. An oversized, yet perfect outfit topper for that chilled office is the ultimate hygge.

2. Street Style Fleece

While athleisure wear still holds the title as the world's most comfortable street style, you can still incorporate loose, soft fabrics into your hygge wardrobe as well. Fleece pants will leave your legs loose and limber with lots of room to stretch and feel fresh air while walking.

3. It is All About the Fabric

Soft knits and neutral hues are, without doubt, the hallmark of hygge. And while the freezing winter months call for an additional layer, there is absolutely no reason why you should abandon these sweaters for the rest of the year.

Hygge Fashion Tips for Men

If you detest being dull and uncomfortable, then it is time to incorporate hygge in your wardrobe. This is because the Danish concept is all about abandoning the slick for cozy knits and baggy jumpers. Thanks to prolonged winter months, staying warm is just the Danes way of life. So borrow a page from their book and hang out in your warmest, comfiest knitwear.

Before you get your eyes rolling, this is not just some flyaway trend. It is also not just another one of those hipster fashions either. Hygge is a Danish concept that comes with anything, and everything, that makes you happy and feeds your soul all year round. It is sort of an answered prayer for folks who hate to shop because they just cannot find anything new.

If you embrace Hygge, you will be taking on the concept of simple living, and that means you will not be chasing after material stuff and flashy possessions. Realizing the ultimate hygge lifestyle is about staying in, curling up with your favorite book or movie, and a cup of coffee – the ultimate life in the slow lane. Along with this, is the choice of effortless outfits that are both comfy and cozy to the extent that you can fall asleep in them.

Here are simple tips to bring more hygge into your wardrobe.

1. Get Knitting

Knitwear is critical when it comes to this Nordic concept. And when it comes to hygge dressing, jumpers (no matter their age), simply do not depreciate. In fact, great knits age like fine wine, appearing more authentic and homely as they begin to show the signs of wear and tear. You can knit your own or get your lovely grandma to make you one.

2. Go for Muted Colors

Remember that shiny "safety jacket" orange shirt that was the "thing" in SS17? Well, how about getting rid of it? That's because the hygge style is all about muted colors. The idea is not to focus all the attention to yourself but rather to blend seamlessly with the surrounding. Much like operating under the radar.

3. Bring the Beanies Back

Beanies will keep your head warm, and that is precisely the point. You really do not want to freeze while out for a walk in the park or with friends for a festive pub crawl. The hygge concept totally respects this. Embrace warmth over style - so grab some gloves, scarves, knitted hats, and beanies. These will be your best allies as long as winter persists, and Dane's way of life is awesome. Match your favorite beanie hat with a pair of geek, simple chic specs and you will have your hygge look nailed.

4. Tight is Not Right

While those slim fit pants will always have a place in your wardrobe, tight shirts and tops are clearly a no-go. Loose fitting and baggy pants are the way to go if you want to embrace hygge.

Hygge Fashion Guide for Ladies

Hygge style is perfect for any season. Think comfortable, not complicated. Cool, but never curated. Cozy, not cold.

Hygge is more than just a trend. It is a way of life that lets you enjoy life's little pleasures.

This could be spending time with loved ones, gathered around the fire with your cups of coffee, reading your favorite book, and riding your bike across town meeting and greeting friends. If you want to get it like the Danes, here are a few tips that can help you incorporate hygge into your wardrobe.

1. Love Everything Knitted

Knitwear is a big deal as far as hygge is concerned. It is the ultimate definition of comfort and coziness and is perfect for keeping warm during those chilly winter months. Keep in mind, hygge is about deriving happiness from the simple things, and that means keeping it practical at all times. The Danes take their health seriously, personal comfort, and well-being ahead of looking cool. Thus, the hygge style is absolutely effortless.

2. *Accessorize for the Weather*

Protection from the elements is critical, both in summer and winter, and Dane's way is by dressing appropriately for the weather. Keeping warm is crucial; scarfs to keep off the cold wind, a hat to protect your head from direct sunlight, and a pair of gloves to protect your skin from cracking.

3. *Protect your Eyes*

Besides protecting your skin from direct sunlight or dry winter air or keeping warm, it is equally important that you protect your eyes. Winter glare can pose a serious health problem, so wearing shades in all seasons is critical. Visit your favorite store for a collection of hygge inspired prescription eyewear and glasses.

4. *Invest in Muted Hues*

Keep it hygge with muted tones to avoid attracting attention to yourself. If adorning all black is not your vibe, consider mixing navy hues, dark greys, deep plums, and browns. The idea is to find subtle shading and a color mix that will blend into any circumstance, whether you are out at night with friends or on a coffee date with someone special.

5. *Give Up the Heels*

Remember, hygge is all about comfort, and that simply means dressing down for pretty much every occasion. The Danes are known for their love for casual dressing in bars and nightclubs. Therefore, comfy trainers and smart, yet casual, outfits are the ultimate looks to pay for. However, if you still love a bit of height, you can replace your stilettos with a pair of your favorite ankle boots. After all, hygge is about comfort and happiness.

CHAPTER 4

HYGGE, FOOD, AND DRINK

Simple Rules for Eating Together the Hygge Way

Hygge, as you probably know by now, is a simple concept of embracing coziness and comfort. Enjoying precious time with loved ones or simply being alone doing what you love. The Danes' focus on hygge is perhaps the main reason why they are considered the happiest people on earth. After all, it is the small things in life that make the difference in the sense of wellbeing.

Candles are not only meant for romantic dinners and blackouts. In fact, they bring so much into life. They are a touch of coziness. So light up the candles. Create an atmosphere of warmth and set the table for a warm meal with friends and family.

Consider creating a team with the family and loved ones. Give everyone a role in making hygge happen. Decide when you are going to have a meal together. Let everyone assume a role, whether it is cooking or just setting up the dinner table. It does not have to be too extravagant. A simple meal is all you need. Just get everyone working together as a team. Have a special evening. Put some thought into presenting the table.

No whining during the hygge dinner. No discussing stresses at work. No negative talk about family, friends, or anyone. Just leave the drama outside and focus on the positive for the evening.

Give up technology. After all, a hygge moment does not have to last hours. Turn off the phones, tablets, computers, and TV while the candles are burning and the meal is getting ready. Gather all the electronics together under a lid and forget about social media for a moment.

Remember that it is about "we" and not "I." Sounds straightforward, right? Well, you might want to think twice. During the hygge moments, do your best to be in touch with the people around you. Stop thinking about your problems and challenges. Ask your company to do the same. Play your favorite game (darts, chase, scrabble, whatever). Share something funny the kids may have said or done.

Focus on those simple things that made you smile and share them. Just an hour or so dedicated to hygge with loved ones after a busy week can reveal to you what you have been missing out on. Of course, it sounds easy; however, it does take practice to reap the benefits.

Suppose Hygge was a Taste, Would it be Kokumi?

To make your food and drinks more hygge-themed, or pleasant, you might want to use kokumi enhancing ingredients. Basically, kokumi is described as the taste that comes from slow-cooked foods rich in flavored gravis. While umami comes with a pleasant, savory taste profile, kokumi delivers a unique basic taste that provides continuity, mouthfulness, and a thick flavor.

Making Room for Imperfection

According to enthusiasts, embracing imperfection is central to living out hygge. Imperfection such as both in your living space and cooking ability, fancy clothing, gourmet food, and formal arrangements have no place in hygge philosophy. Comfort, food, and cozy environments do have their place in hygge philosophy. Remember, the more laid back and intimate, the better.

What this Means

Ditch the fussy canapes and in their place, simmer the soup. Laid-back, comfy things are just the in-thing.

Help your loved ones embrace the imperfections in their own lives. Provide convenient comfort-food options. (You really do not have to prepare a five-course meal). Help your loved ones feel comfortable about appreciating the little moments of joy in their lives. Let them understand that imperfection is ok.

Hygge, Health, Wellness, and Indulgence

Folks are increasingly gravitating towards habitual better-for-life and flavorful treats that make up the critical components of emotionally and physically balanced lifestyles. Same way, hygge envisages both wellness and indulgence. After all, it is all about balance. The point is, incorporating hygge into your life can result in a happier, and thus healthier, life. Hygge, according to USAToday, focuses on the quality of life. Parade describes hygge as one of the hottest trends in health. The New Yorker reports that Danish doctors recommend tea and hygge for the common cold. The Prevention magazine describes hygge as "more than a response to stress..."

What this Means for You

Just find the balance in your life. There is room for convenience, comfort, and indulgence in a well-balanced lifestyle. Remember, too, that hygge is about the wellness of the mind, spirit, and body. That it is all about finding and appreciating those moments of joy and happiness.

Some Takeaways

So, how do you capitalize on hygge in your diet? Well, the point of focus is the balance. After all, part of the appeal of hygge is that it lets you envision moments of peace and tranquility in what would otherwise be a hectic moment. Focus on balance, and help your loved ones do so as well. Perhaps it is a shared meal with a loved one that frees you up to relax. Keep in mind that your loved ones too are attracted to hygge because it gives them room to be imperfect. However, if you choose to incorporate hygge into your kitchen and diet, keep in mind that taste is essential. No matter your flavor, if your food does not inspire love, warmth, and connectedness – it is just not hygge.

CHAPTER 5

HYGGE AND RELATIONSHIPS

The Danes know a thing or two about happiness and contentment. They also know a thing or two about healthy and successful relationships. The Danes made it to the top of the United Nation's World's Happiness Report in 2013, 2014, and 2016. This contentment and happiness can he attributed to hygge – a commitment to coziness, kindness, joy, and overall appreciation of life's little things. At its core, hygge focuses on consciously creating a happy and, satisfied life that extends to relationships.

The hygge principle is a special invisible energy, which is rooted in something between people in a relationship – a unique desire to be together, like a state of mind where you feel connectedness, characterized by proximity, and shared values that transform "I" into "we." Here are just a handful of reasons why the Danes are more satisfied with their relationships than most nationalities.

1. *They Value a Cozy Home*

The Danes, due to the fact that the country experiences extended winter for most of the year, are specifically passionate about creating cozy and happy homes. The Danes are mostly indoors, perhaps because of their hostile weather. Thus, creating a cozy home, that is personal and relaxing, mean a lot to them as far as feeling good is concerned. As they enter their cozy homes, they enter at the same time into a good and lovely energy that makes them happy. When you are happy when you get home, you are likely to find a happy spouse waiting for you.

2. *They Do Not Come Home with the Drama*

Most Danes confess to keeping complaints to a possible minimum and, instead, focusing on positive conversations with their spouses. Of course, that does not mean they never fight. Instead, they are just the opposite of cyborgs. If you want to incorporate hygge into your relationship, then you have to put life's daily dramas under control. Of course, this can be a huge challenge, but when you decide that no negative issues will hold you hostage, then it becomes easier to foster a positive and loving relationship with your spouse.

3. They do not get into debt to fund their weddings

A Danish wedding tends to be a low-key affair, often held in town halls. Also, Danes marry late, at around 35 years for men and 32 years for women, which often means that they have made adequate investments and are financially secure when starting families.

4. Danes are Intentional about the Time They Spend Together

You have probably seen a couple seated together at a dinner and barely talking to one another or walking down the streets in separate bubbles. When the Danes set aside time to be together, they see to it that they truly are together, putting away all distractions to give each other undivided attention.

5. *They Know How to Enjoy the Small Things Together*

Danes love taking pleasure in simple and soothing things. And that is the spirit of hygge. A dinner with a longtime friend is hygge. Large family parties are hygge. The point is, hygge naturally plays into every aspect of Danish life. It is about being kind to the self as well as those close to you that make you a better spouse. Hygge is about being nice to yourself, so you can be nicer to your partner too. This way, the Danes find themselves less spikey to their partners.

6. *They are the Masters of their Own Traditions*

Couples grow stronger together when they are dedicated to implementing certain traditions together. And this, too, is hygge! Shared values can be transformed into life-changing routines that can become traditions when children and loved ones knock on the door.

7. *Their Divorces are Less Nasty*

You are probably wondering why divorce is finding its way in a topic about healthy relationships. Well, to be honest, the way you end a marriage does have a lasting impact. Danes have the fourth highest divorce rates in Europe at 43%. However, their divorces as just as low-key as their weddings. In fact, you can even file your divorce online. Because the female employment is high and social safety is strong, Danish divorces are less likely to turn nasty over money. In fact, a divorce in Denmark can cost you $100 or less. Because divorces are not as acrimonious, there is less stigma attached to them as there is in the U.S. Additionally, most divorced Danes remain friends with some even celebrating their divorce-anniversary over a beer or a well-cooked meal, which is hygge!

Building a Healthy Relationship with Hygge

Here are three C's that can help you embrace hygge and build a fruitful and lasting relationship.

✓ *Communication*

An honest, open dialogue creates room for growth, understanding and eventually, healthy relationships. Open communications and the Danish lifestyle of familiarity and comfort go hand in hand. This is the philosophy of hygge. As you already know, hygge is all about taking your time, slowing down, and freeing yourself from life's hassles. It is about complete dedication to your surroundings and enjoying the present. There can never be a more conducive environment for communication than this.

What is more, healthy communication and hygge creates a positive loop. Hygge creates an environment, a feeling of shared experiences, and harmony, which opens the door for healthy communication. In turn, you develop comfort engaging in meaningful, strong, and inviting feelings of connection and hygge.

How to incorporate hygge in your conversation

Here are a Few Tips

- Switch off distractions like phones and TV and engage fully in the conversation

- Slow down, take your time. There is no point in rushing the discussion

- Open up and share your thoughts as you listen to the other party. Remember, a healthy conversation is a two way traffic

- Be comfortable both mentally and physically. Remember, hygge is all about comfort

- Light up some candles. Remember, it is hygge

✓ *Connection*

If you are observant, you have probably realized the more ways technology connects people, the further apart they get. Guess what: That is not hygge.

Hygge advocates for quality time with loved ones. It is a real conversation while enjoying each other's company. According to Daniel Kahneman's "belongingness hypothesis," every human being has a basic need to relate to others in a close, caring bond. This is an important component of human motivation and behavior. In other words, good relationships equal happy people. That is hygge.

How to Create Hygge Connections

Hygge is humble and slow. It is preferring rustic to new, simple to posh, and tranquility over excitement. So, as you figure out how to connect with loved ones, it is imperative that you keep these values in mind.

- Dress in your hyggelig clothes for a movie night.

- Grab your potluck

- Give up the boardgames. If you live far from the people you love, adapt technology at its finest. You can try out a game night via Skype

- Set up a barbeque or a campfire

- Take a walk or go for a picnic

Feeling Stuck?

So you are trying your best to make these connections but the other party is barely doing their part to meet you halfway? For example, have you planned a hygge night but the other party is simply not having it? Well, no problem. Think about their interests and use the conversation tips discussed above to find out what they would love to do as a team.

They may not be into a camp fire, but how about a game night or some movie?

You may also try to engage in an activity you both love as this can be a great environment for a natural conversation. Plan and prepare dinner together or work on a project or craft that you both enjoy. If these initiatives do not seem to work, you might consider reaching out for help making these connections. There are tons of resources out there that can help you build those relationships.

✓ *Collaboration*

Another important C of hygge living is the collaboration. Hygge is built around chipping in, taking part, and helping out.

Simply put, hygge is all about togetherness.

If you are inviting friends over for dinner, for instance, it is ok…in fact it is great if you asked for help fixing the dinner. You can also take it a step further to make it a potluck. This way, everyone gets to share in the experience. Remember, it is more hyggeligt if everyone participates in food preparation, instead of leaving everything to the host.

Similarly, if you are sharing stories or are engaged in conversations, be sure to listen as much as (if not more) than you talk. Collaboration, Equality, and shared experiences are the building blocks of hygge. It is important that everyone has room in the conversation.

So as you move towards building healthy, lasting relationships, creating time for loved ones, and practicing work-life balance, never get hygge philosophy out of mind. Learn to practice engaged conversations by participating in activities that build connections, and build togetherness through collaboration.

11 Helpful Ways to Practice Hygge as a Family

There are multiple ways to embrace hygge as a family, but here are a few practical ways you can get the whole family to embrace hygge.

Decide to Make it a Point, Not an Accident

First, hygge does not come naturally. It is made to happen. With a long to-do list (from homework to house chores) setting time aside to practice hygge is deliberate. You, the adult, will need to decide if and when you want to hygge. Evenings are great times to get together and have some hygge moment. You may want to set aside 30 minutes to one hour a week to have great times with your loved ones. If evening hygge is already part of your lifestyle, well done!

Create Comfortable Meeting Places

Comfort is a major component of hygge. This means everyone may not want to sit on a hard floor to play some board game. Get together pillows, pallets, blankets, and stuffed animals and create some comfort.

Go Technology Free

Technology is great. However, it can be a major source of distraction. They have a way of pulling people to the "urgent," which is genuinely not as urgent, and you are left feeling empty and guilty for the time it took you away from loved ones. If you are going to embrace hygge, then be sure to switch off your phones, tablets, computers, and the television, unless you are watching a movie.

Be in the Present

One of the biggest goals of hygge is to build a bond between people. Your loved ones are your people, and in order to maximize the time together, be sure to focus on them. This is why you need to be in the present. Learn to listen, ask questions, and give answers. In short, just learn to be you.

Without trying to modify anyone's thoughts, moods and behavior, try to encourage an environment of ambiance. Hygge is about relaxing and managing the entire situation. It may sound easy to do, but it's actually quite hard to do.

Cook Together

An important hygge rule of thumb: the longer it takes to prepare a meal, the better. Hygge foods are soups, stews, comfort food, and of course, lovely company. Hygge time should set aside the normal dietary restrictions while letting you embrace what you love the most.

What tastes great? What is fun to prepare? And what is handmade? That is hygge. Remember, when it comes to hygge and food, rustic is better than prissy. Chunky and hearty sweets or snacks are far better than souffles, quiches, and macaroons. Hygge is all about hassle free comfort.

Play Board Games

Board games are an excellent way to bond over shared activities. Of course, this may be hard to do when your kids are small, but there are still some board games that you can get preschoolers to play. For instance, you can get together with your friends once a month to play Axis and Allies, a game that can take you through 14 hours! Sharing warm drinks, food, and several hours of long board games can create epic memories that will last for years to come.

Check Out those Old Photos

Hygge seeks to inspire a warm, fuzzy feeling. Nothing can be better than crawling up on the couch with a cup of coffee while traveling back in time browsing through your kid's baby photos with them. How about taking your kids through your own baby photos? This is a perfect way to get everyone hooked. You will refresh your memory with things you have not thought through in months, and your kids will be pleased to see where they, or you, came from and how you have all got to where you are. There is nothing as homey as this, and this is the spirit of hygge.

Wear Comfortable Clothes

You can never have a hyggelig evening in a pair of tight, restrictive jeans. If you have friends and family around, you are better off nixing the pajamas. And when hygging as a family, consider changing into your pajamas, yoga pants, sweats, comfortable socks, and a pair of slippers. In other words, feel comfortable and relaxed.

Woolen socks are recommended for their incredible warmth and comfort. You can also get soft robes for your evening wear since they feel nice, are cozy, and generally prettier than the basic pajamas. After a shower, when everyone has wet hair, is the perfect time sit back for precious hygge moments.

Get Hot Drinks

There is nothing like a hot, or warm, drink to create a cozy environment. If you have little ones around, consider preparing for them warm milk mixed with melted chocolate or cocoa powder. Kids love chocolate milk.

57

The concept of warmth and comfort is key to hygge, so a chilled Diet Coke may not be ideal for cozying up. You can prepare drinks on the crock pot or stove, and preparing the drinks itself is a perfect way to experience hygge in the evening.

Do Not Prepare the Agenda

Hygge moment is not the time to discuss the family's financial situation or read the riot's act to a friend or a loved one. It is not the time to point out your kid's unbecoming behaviors. In short, it is not the time to bring up topics that raise anxiety. It is time to sit back and bond as a family. Therefore, be sure to pay attention to everyone's flow. If your kids want to play board games, let them go ahead. Or better yet, join them. If they enjoy lying with you on the bed reading their story books, tag along.

Doing hygge as a family requires very few goals. And here are some of them:

- To give everyone a sense of security and safety

- To create a cozy and homey environment

- To strengthen the family bond

How you get to these is entirely up to you, but it is important that you do it.

Hygge and Parenting

There is a growing fascination with the Danes' way of life, and here is the reason...

You probably know the dangers of modern life's plugged-in, isolated culture when it comes to families and relationships. Countless books have been written about the dangers of modern technology. However, it is not the technology that is standing between people and happiness; this is just the latest escape route. What people really need to do is slow down and embrace the various inputs and outputs that life brings along, giving relationships time to flourish.

Most people never slow down. They just bring in new inputs (the latest efficiency application or life hacker) that make them more productive and efficient, but that does not really slow down their minds or make any significant improvement to their lifestyles and relationships. This is the typical American way of confronting a problem, which is in part responsible for the current trend of fascination with the Danes' philosophies of life.

Here are practical tips that can help you incorporate hygge and parent like the Danes.

1. Encourage your children to be independent. You can achieve this by introducing regular independent activities throughout the day.

2. Intentionally set aside time in the day to spend with your kids

3. Build your discipline approach on mutual respect rather than on fear and punishment

4. Regularly schedule a time to unplug and exercise hygge as a family.

These concepts are quite easy to implement and they are not magic bullets.

Independence is Important for Children

Kids can never successfully grow under the intimidating presence of an overprotective dad or mom. Of course, the average parent does not choose to be overprotective, but it is quite easy to fall into the habit. Encouraging kids to be independent can be difficult. It makes menial chores take about 30 times longer than what is important when parents just handle them for their kids.

It is not always easy, but it is important to take your time and let the kids learn how to handle things on their own. It is also absolutely possible for a kid to play and entertain him or herself. Independent play is a great opportunity for a child to learn essential life skills, develop their creativity, and develop both cognitively and physically.

Encouraging Intentional Time

Telling a child "no" when he or she asks to do things alongside you may seem harsh. But it is not a final "no," it is just a "no" for the moment. When children know that they can play or work on their own, they will learn to concentrate more on their tasks and develop vital life skills. They will no longer be desperate for their attention, and this is vital for independence.

There is the temptation to build independence in the child, and then keeping off intentional time. It can get ugly. Kids may not want to play or function alone (or even use the toilet by themselves) because they badly want to spend time with you. So, even if it is just movie or reading time at night, or if they can join hands with you in the kitchen, it is a step in the right direction towards Hygge. Set time to bond with your kids – just you and them, without the risk of reaching for your phone.

A Regular Sabbath is Essential

Admittedly, most families are poor at this one. The Sabbath idea goes way back to the ancient Jewish concept of prayer, rest, and reflection. For 24 hours, starting Friday through to Saturday, Jews do not work. They rest and pray. Their week hinges on this. Of course, you do not have to follow this verbatim, but you can plan some pocket of time and leisure. Genuine leisure though, not resigning into couch potato mode. Laziness will only make exhaustion worse.

The most important aspect of Sabbath is finding a way of incorporating peace and silence. This usually means forgetting those pesky phone calls and staying away from social media to put together some sanity.

But, it is more than just giving technology a break. It is about unplugging from technology in order to plug into the community. This is where hygge, the magic sauce to the happy Danish home comes in. Read a novel out loud as a family over some hot coffee. Grab the sleeping bags and sleep under the sky, stargazing over cups of hot coffee. Pick up and play a long board game that extends for hours. Whatever makes you tick, get some rest. Even if it is a Monday or Friday night, it really does not matter when or for how long, it is important that you spare time for leisure and rest. That is the spirit of hygge.

The points to note here are not that you have to become Danish or stress out if you are not perfectly doing all the things mentioned above. However, implementing a thing or two will hopefully get your otherwise hectic household to slow down and relax.

CHAPTER 6

HYGGE THROUGHOUT THE YEAR

Hygge can vary from person to person. That is, what is hygge to one may be boring or irrelevant to another. For instance, if you are a landscaper, chances are you will be looking for ways to make your clients happy and fulfilled. It will surprise you that you are inherently incorporating hygge into your work and life all year round.

Hygge for Winter

Depending on where you are, winter can be darker, colder, and more hostile than the rest of the year. While winter is typically a down time for most activities, Holidays tend to be the peak time for hygge. This is the most hygge-like or hyggelig time of the year. During holidays, the Danes tend to decorate their homes and streets with green, red, and gold lights.

This is the perfect time of the year to embrace togetherness and unity of purpose. Outdoor lighting, spa tubs, fire pits, and landscape lighting make just about any winter more hygge.

Professional companies offer holiday lighting that keeps families and loved ones warm and safe indoors. The bright lights stand out in sharp contrast to the long, gloomy winter nights. Seeing these lights bring warmth and ignite the spirit of hygge throughout the holiday season.

Fire pits are just the ideal hygge accessory for winter. Grab your woolen basket, a glass of wine, your loved one, and spend the evening gazing at the stars.

Hot tubs or spas? One of the greatest hygge feelings you will experience is a moment at the hot tub or spa. It gets better when you are with a loved one. To the Danes, hygge is the hallmark of the cold season. And with the long, dark winter, they genuinely need it.

Hygge and Spring

Most people consider Spring as the least hygge season. However, it may be hygge in itself as it is a welcome break after a brutal winter.

Leaves and blooms reappear, offering a much-needed welcome from an unforgiving winter. Birds start singing, the sun reappears, and the snow melts away leaving a nostalgic earth behind.

Bulbs planted during fall make for spectacular, aromatic cut flowers to give any home the interior feel of hygge. Proximity to nature is an essential component of hygge to pretty much everyone.

Creating a community garden makes for an excellent Earth Day project. Not to mention, it is a great opportunity to get together as a community and build a lasting relationship.

If you find this endeavor inviting, you may consider joining a community garden that is already established or is simply plant some pollinator friendly plants you will enjoy in summer.

Hygge and Summer

As already mentioned over and over, hygge is all about appreciating and finding pleasure in life's simple things. Fresh air, a warm sunshine, fireplaces, barbeques, a soft grass, picnics, cookpots, and yard games are just a few things that come with this season.

Water features, patios, outdoor kitchens, and fire pits, are all simple features that can contribute towards bringing the hygge concept to your home.

Not just any patio will be ideal. The secret is in the design. If you include a seating wall, be sure to arrange such so that people can sit close to and enjoy the company of each other.

Make outdoor kitchens spacious enough so that families and guests can participate in meal preparation. You can use brick ovens for creating a rustic pizza. This is a great way of bringing people together as they participate in creating their own comfort food.

Accent fire pits should be with comfortable seating that features cushions, blankets, and pillows. Most important, always encourage comfort food – from hot-dogs to marshmallows. There should be no dieting or deprivation when it comes to hygge.

Water features can be naturalistic or contemporary, but they should come with that therapeutic sound of peace.

A summer solstice bonfire is an excellent addition when you want to host an event with a few of your intimate family and friends.

Create tranquil "hyggakrog" or nooks in your landscapes that are conducive for book reading, hammock laying, or simply taking nature treks.

Another simple way to incorporate hygge into your summer is to host an outdoor movie night. All you need to make this happen is a project, a white sheet, and an audience, of course.

Hygge and Autumn

True autumn is a wonderful season for hygge. The feeling you get when you come back home after raking the leaves, and kick back with a warm cider or a hot cup of coffee, that is hygge.

A walk through the yard or flower garden, enjoying the colors before the leaves fall off, that too is hygge.

A well thought-out outdoor landscaping and lighting offers a great glimmer of hope as the colder, darker months approach by illuminating your home's welcoming features and your landscape's texture. You may want to invest in professionally installed low-voltage systems. Besides being eco-friendly, they also improve your home's safety, browser security, and landscape.

Most people make the mistake of choosing landscape lights without considering how they look from the inside.

Lighting up your backyard or tree can make a huge difference when the dark, winter months approach.

The Danes love the lighting. Like landscapers, lighting to them is pretty much an art.

Hassle-Free Hygge Ideas for the Year

One of the toughest, yet simple ways, to incorporate hygge in your home is to opt for phone-free times. Disconnecting from the world and connecting to the family is a surefire way of building a closer, stronger family.

Year-long candles are a beautiful way to bring hygge into your home. Danes love unscented candles that do not have artificial elements. These can be incorporated both indoors and outdoors. Just remember to blow them out when done.

You may swap out light bulbs to warmer hues in order to mimic sunrise or sunset while giving your home a cozy feel.

Host outdoor or indoor game nights or craft beer exchanges.

Finally, always remember when decorating or hosting that casual is important. A casual environment creates ambiance and serenity.

So, whether you are evaluating your indoor and outdoor space, be sure to find ways to make them more hygge.

CHAPTER 7

HYGGE AND THE WORKPLACE

Are you busy and stressed? According to surveys, up to 90 percent of employees admit stress in the workplace. So, chances are your co-workers are equally stressed as well. Whether you are chasing a tough deadline, struggling to strike a realistic work-life balance, or walking up two hours ahead of everyone else to snow-blow the driveway, you can find a way to incorporate hygge in your workplace, too.

The concept of hygge is gaining popularity in the workplace. Here are some simple tips that can help you introduce a little hygge to your workplace.

1. Power in Numbness

While you can opt to have your lunch at your desk and catch up with your social media networks, hygge encourages a sense community and togetherness. Grab your lunch with workmates or participate in an all-staff event when called upon. According to the International Founding finding on Workplace Wellness, 57% of employers offer some form of onsite celebrations or events while 45% of employers provide staff outings.

2. Practice Mindfulness in the Workplace

Certainly, this is easier said than done. Taking a minute or two to refill your water bottle, as well as mingling with colleagues, goes a long way in promoting the spirit of hygge at the workplace. Also, make use of the meditation or yoga facility at your workplace.

3. Take Coffee Time Seriously

For an instant hygge, why not grab some warm, cozy coffee, tea, or chocolate. According to surveys, 62 percent of employers offer a coffee break.

Hygge tip: Bring your joy sparking mug to the workplace and keep the excitement flowing along with the coffee.

4. *Shower Your Workspace with Some Love*

Be sure to have a handful of photos of people and things you really love. Some artwork that makes you relax, a pen organizer, a small plant or an accent lamp if you have space for it. The point is, declutter what you should and make your workspace as hygge friendly as you can.

5. *Be Nice*

Friendliness and companionship are vital components of hygge. You do not have to go full Pollyanna but think of ways you can make the workplace fun and friendly for your team. Offer a hand to a frazzled colleague. Say good morning even if you are barely in the mood. Buy someone a cup of coffee. Be the colleague everyone is proud to work alongside…because that is the concept of hygge.

Even if You Live in a Warm Climate, You can still Embrace Hygge.

It is easy to maintain the attitude of comfort, security, and well-being when you are at home surrounded by laughter and a cup of great coffee, warm socks, candlelight, homemade snacks, and beautiful flowers. The workplace is the one place where everyone needs hygge the most. The last thing you want is to show up at your workplace moping and looking drowsy from lack of motivation. You want to greet your workmates with kindness and excitement for the day ahead.

Your workplace is the ideal place to embrace this Danish concept. Here are seven ways to entrench the culture of hygge in your workplace.

1. Come to Work with Your Mug

Nothing is more relaxing than sipping a warm beverage even during the hot summer days. Caffeine is a great way to boost your energy levels and ensure that you are focused on your work. Take time to enjoy your cup of coffee with colleagues as you chat about non-work-related issues. Just keep off politics and other sensitive topics. And don't forget that bringing your favorite mug to the workplace is pretty much like carrying a piece of home with you. Do not be afraid to refill as you take a break from mundane tasks.

2. Create a Relaxing Work Playlist

Nothing relaxes the mind like good music. Make up an upbeat, yet calming playlist, like acoustic tunes, that get you through your workday. Take advantage of services like Spotify and iTunes to create a hygge playlist that will get you up and running through the day.

3. Have Your Lunch Outside or Take Some Time to Unwind with Colleagues

When it is a lunch break, do take the BREAK! This is not the time to check your mails, stare at your computer, or plan for your afternoon task while eating the lunch you carried from home. Instead, it is the time to step outside and enjoy some fresh air. Depending on the location of your workplace, take a walk around the block or across the street to their nearest deli and enjoy your lunch with colleagues at the park. Whatever you opt for, stepping out of the office will help you catch some fresh air and rejuvenate yourself in readiness for your next assignment.

4. Decorate Your Desk or Workspace

It is ok to decorate your workspace with personal items like a family picture or a bouquet of tulips that you bought at the farmer's market over the weekend. Having vintage books stacked around your desk can be great too. Just be sure not to cross the company policy's red line or clutter your desk. Whatever you do, make your workspace a comfortable, special haven that inspires you to be productive. You can also give your office a cozier feel with artwork, a cozy chair, and sentimental items that define your personal life.

5. Organize a Potluck with Coworkers

Comfort food is the basis of all things hygge. There is no better way to savor home-cooked meals than with your workmates by your side taste-testing your meals. That is hygge. The point is, eating together sets the stage to hygge with colleagues. This way, you get to connect and enjoy relaxed moments together. You may also organize a potluck day rather than carrying your lunch from home. Remember, when everyone shares, everyone partakes in the spirit of hygge.

6. Embrace Random Acts of Kindness for Your Colleagues

Whether you are carrying to your workplace a box of cookies or simply extending a compliment to a colleague, you will turn someone's day as well as your own around with a simple act of kindness. That is the spirit of hygge.

7. Embrace Teamwork

Team spirit is very much at the center of Danish culture. Right from childhood, Danes learn to work as a team and are taught to seek and/or help each other in the face of adversity. They are empowered to hold on to their confidence and humility despite their strengths and weaknesses.

8. *Learn to be Calm and Content*

Hygge, unlike the physical stuff that you can create or touch, is a state of mind. With stress being one of the top causes of employee absenteeism, the workplace should offer calming features that take the pressure off when deadlines are looming.

Consider taking advantage of those quirky office perks, those lunchtime yoga classes, or meditation sessions to calm down. Homemade sweets and cookies are also an important part of the Danish concept of hygge, so why not organize, say weekly or monthly, office food rotations where the teams will take turns to cook and carry homemade cookies to the office? Remember, hygge is all about creating a soothing environment devoid of chaos. So, be sure to make the workplace as relaxed as possible.

The spirit of cooperation and teamwork is exhibited in pretty much every aspect of the Danish life – right from the classroom, to the workplace, as well as in family life. Seeing the family or colleagues work as a team develops a strong sense of belonging. You can take the same concept to the boardroom as well.

You can organize team building events like scavenger hunt contests to encourage the spirit of working together. Once you embrace hygge at the workplace, you will start appreciating those small and special moments that really matter in life.

The Hygge décor and Your Workplace: The Employer's Role

Hygge is about creating the ideal environment that gives your staff the security they need while ensuring that they are both creative and productive. With the approval of your health and safety team, you can introduce candles to add to the ambiance of the workplace. No one enjoys sitting under the fluorescent light all day long, so consider how lighting can improve your employee's look and feel.

Design too is critical. Wood has a special way of giving Danes a homely feel, so if possible be sure to incorporate wood into the design of your workplace.

Think about alternatives to the traditional rows and computer desks. Try mixing it up a little in order to create a sense of community based on the seating plan where team leaders get to mix with their teams. Separate partitioning for purposes of demarcating ranks or positions is very much anti-hygge.

Create more homely spaces with communal seating and sofas for activities that can be shared with the entire team such as brainstorming or meeting sessions.

Hot desking negates the idea of hygge. However, if you have to include it in your office culture, be sure to seek your employees' ideas when designing hot desks, so they can occupy desired areas based on their moods.

Finally, encourage employees to come and bring their own mugs and personal pictures to create workspaces that help them feel comfortable and happy in the office.

Smart Casual is Cool...

Designs go beyond the interiors. Uniforms are anything but hygge. The reason? They do not let people be themselves or feel at ease. On the contrary, dress down days is very much hygge. In fact, the smart casual dressing is quite a bang.

Hygge: The Culture of Togetherness

Studies have proven that one of the most essential ingredients to happiness is hanging around other people, especially the people with whom you have a connection with. Workplace camaraderie is crucial, so figure out how to create opportunities that bring your employees together and build in as strong teams as possible.

Create an environment where your team members can work remotely from home. Some people would not mind working from home, especially during those dark winter months.

Encourage video calls through skype instead of email and phone calls at least once in a day. However, this should not be a substitute for physical contact. It is important that you hold regular and physical meetings with your staff for updates. An occasional team lunch would also be a great option.

Make Hygge the Frame of Mind...

Studies have shown that self-critical people tend to have low mental health and life satisfaction levels. Naturally, everyone needs to reflect on their skillset and make deliberate efforts to improve. No one benefits from focusing on the negative. Being content with your current situation and your role at the workplace is of critical importance, and it is up to your team leader to ensure you derive fulfillment from your work.

Like a bad apple amongst fresh ones, an eternal pessimist can truly dent the mood in the workplace. The negativity can spread through like wild fire, shredding productivity in its wake. Every employee's wellbeing is critical to ensure hygge thrives in the workplace.

Hygge during Lunchtime

Everyone needs a break. If your team leader scowls at your vacant desk during the designated lunch break, they should take a closer look at their leadership style.

Taking a break boosts your productivity for the rest of the day, so it is a false economy clinging to your desk hoping to win points from your team leader.

Here, team leaders need to take a critical look at the process and results of every individual's output during a working day rather than the amount of time it takes to complete an assignment.

Lunch times are also perfect for getting the team together, enjoying their food while discussing current issues with colleagues, which all contributes to a friendly and productive working environment.

Hygge at Home, Happy at the Work

If your team members and their families are happy at home, it is very likely they will also carry that happiness to the workplace. Of course, this is not to suggest that you ram hygge down their throats, but if you are promoting the culture of hygge in the workplace, then you may want to discuss it with your team about the possibility of adopting the concept in their homes as well.

It is up to your staff to find out more about hygge and how they can introduce the concept into their homes.

Hygge Treats

Besides being the happiest people in the world, Danes are also the biggest consumers of sugar and sweet treats. You may not hear the saying "add a little sugar to your life," but providing Danish pastries and cookies to the workplace once a week can go a long way in lifting everyone's spirit in the office.

CHAPTER 8

HYGGE ON A BUDGET

You have probably seen those memes that articulate how life in Denmark is beautiful, right? Well, Danes are happy people, and hygge has something to do with it. And the best part is, you do not have to pay through the nose to incorporate hygge into your life. Here is how you can incorporate hygge in your shopping budget.

1. Clearly Understand What You Need

What do you need to feel enough hygge in your home and life? What are you yearning for? For most people, warmth and comfort are paramount. In this case, you may want to get some woolen socks, lots of coffee (or tea), and wrap up in plenty of scarves. With a clear understanding of what you want, or what you think will make you incorporate hygge into your life, you are more likely to find fulfillment.

2. *Buy Used Items*

You do not have to buy brand new designer items to feel cozy or embrace hygge. Why spend hundreds of dollars on new furniture when you can get used ones for less? Check your local store or look up on Craigslist for used arm chairs, couches, blankets, and even clothing.

Point to note: hygge is not about being frugal. Rather, it is about being content.

3. *Shop at the Discount Store*

Have you ever stopped by the Marshalls' sales section? It is the one place in a store that draws most folks. You could buy everything from this section if you have space and money. From blankets to pillows, to candles, to snacks, you can get pretty much everything here. The best part is that their products are more affordable than they would otherwise be. So, check out the discount section in your local store. You never know how much you will save on discounts. However, be sure not to indulge in impulsive buying.

4. Create a Hygge Fund

If you feel you need to make some upgrades in your home or life, but cannot afford it presently, save up! Consider opening a saving fund that is specifically meant for hygge-ing your life. You may want to do a little homework to know how much you will need to pay for the items you are envisioning. You may automate the savings from your salary and use a savings application to set aside the proper amount to save.

5. Start with One Hygge Space

Sometimes, you are better off starting small. This is specifically important when you are making overarching changes to your home and lifestyle. To make your hygge dream a reality, choose one component of you home to start with. This could be the cozy corner in your living room or the reading nook in your bedroom. Perhaps you want your next winter clothing to be a little bit softer and warmer. Identify one priority area to get started. Remember, hygge is about happiness and contentment. You do not have to rush things.

Simple Tips to Hygge on a Budget

Stay at Home

The primary concept of hygge is in its simplicity and affordability. So stay indoors! Do not step out into the biting winter cold. Hygge simply means getting to enjoy the comfort of your own home, saving the money that you would otherwise spend on expensive drinks or Uber rides. Invite your family or friends over and spend the day hygge-ing together while building long lasting memories.

Include a Flagship Mug in Tour Collection

You really do not need the minimalist design Danish leather couch to be fully hygge. Rather, you can spend as little as $20 on a mug that will bring you joy and fulfillment with each use. The only catch is it must eventually become your favorite mug, one that warms your heart every time you sip your coffee from it.

Embrace Fire

You do not have to be a pyromaniac or anything. However, if you have an open fireplace, then you need to dust it off. Light up the candles too. Imagine you are in a log cabin up in the mountains just by yourself. Grab your cup of coffee and your favorite book. Turn on some slow music. Kick back and relax. That is hygge.

Get crafty

Learn an art. Knit, sew, or glue gun and craft things together to make yourself beanies, socks, pillowcases, sweaters, blankets, or just about any artwork that comes to mind. Anything that will add coziness to your living space is also hygge.

Read more

The philosophy of hygge lies not in having to do much to experience hygge. Go through your book collection and spend the chilly winter months indoors reading through your favorite books.

Do not give up cooking delicious meals

Bring your family and friends into the kitchen and start baking. Make homemade cookies, bread, cakes, or muffins and enjoy while they are still warm. Soup is to hygge as what fuel is to a car, and rustic, homemade meals are the foundation on which a healthy hygge lifestyle is built upon. Save money on restaurants and start cooking your own food at home instead. You will be amazed at how the whole family will be brought together by a well cooked meal.

Find indulgence in small pleasures

Hygge is about deriving pleasures from the simple things in life, not the expensive things. Cuddle up with the one you love at night, run a steaming hot bubble bath, pop up some popcorn, or watch your favorite movies. The point is, appreciate the little things that give you the feeling of warmth and fullness both in and out.

CHAPTER 9

GETTING STARTED WITH HYGGE

So you have read everything there is about hygge and you want to get started with it right away? Well, here is how you can start introducing this Danish philosophy into your way of life.

Start Taking Time Out

In a world where everyone is busy, it is easy to forget to reflect and appreciate the moment you are in. Studies show that every American spends about 5 hours per day on their smartphone. Think about the first thing you do as soon as you wake up. For most folks, it is grabbing their phones to check out their emails or social media accounts. Interestingly, this is also the last thing most folks do before retiring to bed. It is also the same thing they do while on their way to work, at the dinner table, and just about everywhere else! The result is information overload, leaving you with barely enough room to breathe and appreciate the beauty of life or build lasting bonds with loved ones. This is where the concept of hygge comes in. Start by cutting back on the amount of time you spend with your smartphone, computers, and other forms of technology. Instead, dedicate more time to self-love, time with family and friends, and relaxation doing the things you love.

Think Introvert

To most people, hygge is the "introvert's answer to a great time." Perhaps this could be true with the Danes. It is widely known that the Danes are the happiest humans in the world. In fact, Danes are ranked among the top 5 happy nationalities. While multiple factors contribute to happiness and that happiness is not possible to measure, you should reckon that being at peace with yourself is key to being happy. The Danes are excellent at it! You can start embracing hygge by creating time for yourself.

Hygge is a feeling of peace of mind, warmth, a sense of belonging, wellbeing, and appreciation of the moment.

Unfortunately, this is what many introverts struggle to achieve. The society exerts too much pressure on introverts to fit in and interact in the workplace or in groups, forgetting that not everyone is wired for this lifestyle. Some introverts make the mistake of giving in to fit in only to discover that true happiness and contentment comes from deep within. The key to hygge lies in learning how to appreciate and enjoy your own company and the company of the people that you care about. This is the concept of hygge.

Embracing the Hygge Self

Hygge does not come with definite rules or dos and don'ts that make the concept appealing. It is about appreciating the little joys of everyday living according to your taste and preferences. You are not bound by stringent rules. Rather, hygge encourages you to live your life in the simplest possible form. You might be living hygge life without even realizing it. For instance, if you have ever stayed out at night by the fireplace warming up with a cup of coffee and your favorite book, or spent the whole day indoors wrapped up in your blanket, or light up the candle, then you have already had a taste of hygge life. All you need to do is create a lifestyle out of these.

If you are an introvert, embracing a hygge life may simply mean dedicating more time to enjoying your company, and spending quality with loved ones creating lasting memories.

Simplicity is Key

Hygge emphasizes owning less. A hygge life is characterized by minimalism. While it does not teach you to give up all your possessions, you would probably appreciate that it is the extras you own or wish you owned that distracts you from appreciating what you presently own. Hygge also prefers that rustic home-made stuff over factory made. You can ditch your bedside lamp for a candlelight, or give up your designer sweater for cozy, hand-made alternatives. So, you'll want to start by decluttering and simplifying your life as much as you can.

It is the Little Pleasures

Hygge advocates enjoying what you simply love. You need to start by identifying those things and hygge does not call for trying too much. That means trial and error is out! The idea is finding a meeting point between what makes you happy and the contentment of enjoying the little daily pleasures that are special to you. Furthermore, hygge can be experienced both indoors and outdoors. Enjoying a bike ride with a group of friends or taking a morning jog with your puppy is also hygge. After all, the key to hygge is deriving comfort and fulfillment in being yourself and cherishing life's simple, yet precious, moments. There is really no need to over think or exaggerate anything. Simply do what makes you happy. No need to fit into some philosophy or please anyone.

Create time for friends and family

Togetherness is an important aspect of hygge. Spending quality time with the people you cherish is a great way to kick start your hygge, and it does not really matter what you do. A dinner party, a morning or evening jog, a coffee date, or even a Netflix binge is all you need to do the trick.

Multi-Tasking is Against the Spirit of Hygge

Hygge is all about finding fulfillment, and that means multi-tasking is out. If you find yourself turning on your computer, or grabbing your phone to check your work emails while watching a movie with friends or family then know that you are breaking one of the very few hygge rules.

If you keep drifting out of a conversation with your spouse to clean the dishes, stop. Appreciate the time with your spouse and try to steer the conversation towards a subject matter that most of you are interested in. Hygge is a time to focus on enjoying your leisure without feeling bad about it.

Leave Work at a Reasonable Time

Danes have a strong belief in a healthy work-life balance. As a matter of fact, they emphasize it. They do not appreciate long working hours, and their parental leave policy (which is 52 weeks) is incredibly generous. It is no wonder that Denmark ranks high on the list of countries with the best work-life balance.

So, if you want to copy Dane's way of life, start by leaving work at a reasonable time. Of course, it is important that you accomplish your daily work targets. That said, stop lingering behind to score some points with your boss or stay around working on the following day's assignment.

Go home and get cozy instead.

Eat Well

Food is an integral part of the hygge. In fact, the whole idea of hygge lifestyle is also described as "healthy hedonism." It is not healthy hedonism if fine food and good drinks are not in the equation.

There is no guilty in hygge. Just a huge bowl of winter salads, almond cake, or spiked punch. It works best when you prepare your own food at home. No eating out!

Wear Comfortable Outfits

Hygge advocates for constant comfort. If you want round-the-clock comfort, you will need to dress for it. However, this does not mean you have to put on dowdy sweats through the winter months. Refer to the section on incorporating hygge into your wardrobe for some tips. It works best when you ditch your designer labels for simple, home knitted sweaters.

CONCLUSION

Gathering by the firepot on a dark, cold night, lighting up the candles, wearing a home-made woolly sweater, sipping hot coffee or mulled wine, and petting your puppy – that is certainly hygge.

Munching home-made popcorns. Cuddling up on the couch. Watching movies with friends and family. Enjoying a hot cup of tea. Family reunion at Christmas. All these are hygge. Pronounced "hoo-ga," this Danish word loosely translates into "coziness", but it is much more than just that. Hygge is an attitude to life that makes one learn to appreciate and derive love, happiness, and satisfaction from life's simple gifts.

BONUS

As you already know, Hygge is about comfort, coziness, and simplicity. It's a way of living. It promotes minimalism and staying organized. I wanted to elaborate on this. That's why I created an ebook called *Getting Yourself Organized*. It's a collection of tips that can help you stay more organized and declutter your house. It's completely free. To receive it, just type the link below into your browser and download your book.

https://bit.ly/2PCx0wO